# THE

# FOAM ROLLER

# BIBLE

FOAM ROLLING

SELF MASSAGE, TRIGGER POINT
THERAPY & STRETCHING

*Second Edition*

CHASE WILLIAMS

© 2015

## COPYRIGHT NOTICE

## DISCLAIMER

This book is not intended as a substitute for the medical advice of physicians. The reader should regularly consult a physician in matters relating to his/her health and particularly with respect to any symptoms that may require diagnosis or medical attention.

# CONTENTS

# INTRODUCTION

While foam rolling has been around for quite a while, until recently it's been mostly a mysterious technique used by professional athletes, coaches, and therapists to help increase mobility and overall muscle tone.

These days, however, it can be found in gyms, on T.V. and in homes across the nation, with more people seeing the benefits of foam rolling every day.

The problem is, while most people have seen and heard of Foam Rolling, many still do not know how to use it or what it's even supposed to do. Unless you have your very own therapist trained in foam rolling techniques, or you are a professional athlete with a guru teaching you the methods and benefits of foam rolling, you probably also have many questions pertaining to foam rolling, as well. I assume that's the reason you are reading this book now.

That's the reason I wrote this book. To show the average Joe (or Jolene) the best possible methods for Foam Rolling, right in your own home. You would probably pay a professional hundreds of dollars for what you will learn in this book and even then they probably still won't even teach you half of what you will discover herein. Not only will you learn the best exercises for foam rolling, but you will also learn what these exercises do and why you should be using them.

I have tried my best to keep the language in this book easy to understand, and stayed away from the more "specialty" words, such as medical jargon and technical terms. Where such words and language are used, I've tried to explain them in an easy to understand manner. If you do come across something in this book you simply cannot understand, I highly recommend you look it up on line to increase your knowledge and understanding.

To start off with, this book will introduce you to a brief history of the foam roller and how it came to be such an integral part of many peoples lives today. You'll discover just why so many people seem to be drawn to this simple foam rolling device and why so many athletes, coaches and trainers are beginning to incorporate it into their practice.

From there you'll learn just what myofascial release is all about and how it pertains to these rolling exercises. Although self myofascial release may sound like so much technical gobbledygook, you'll find here that (as it pertains to foam rolling) it's more or less just a fancy way of saying "self massage". We'll discuss what the fascia is and how it works, as well as how to release fascial adhesions (or knots), so that you are not just doing the exercises but you know

WHY these exercises are helping you, which is always a plus.

If you are a runner, we've included a chapter about why foam rolling should be a vital part of your running routine and why stretching exercises alone may not be enough, indeed they may even be detrimental if you are stretching prior to running. By utilizing foam rolling, you can help keep your ligaments and muscles from becoming stiff and rigid as well as minimizing trigger points that often come from overworked muscles.

Another area we will touch upon in this book is incorporating foam rolling into your yoga routine. You'll find that by incorporating the foam roller into the many different yoga poses you can achieve a much better result than you would by simply doing the yoga poses by themselves. We will discuss how to do this as well as give a few examples to get you started.

Toward the end of this book you'll find how foam rolling can not only make you feel much better and increase your mobility, but also aid in staving off many age-related ailments such as arthritis and bursitis and other problems that are all-to-often chalked up to "your just getting old". We'll discuss how you can even reverse the effects of some ailment by rolling on a regular basis.

I've also included a brief description of the many different foam rollers available to help you decided on the one that's perfect for you, if you haven't already got one yourself. I do recommend, however, that if you are just beginning in foam rolling you go with the softer more pliable foam rollers. Once you have been rolling for a while, you can move on to the firmer (and often more painful) rollers out there.

I highly recommend you read all the way through this book and don't skip any of the earlier chapters, as a background on the rollers and self-myofascial release will help tremendously in understanding these exercises and how they can help you in different ways. You can, of course, choose to skip over the brief history, but you may find it fascinating, or at the very least educational, so the next time you are the gym you can show off your above-average knowledge.

Even if you are not a professional athlete, you will find foam rolling can be of much benefit in your daily workout. It can help you before and after exercises and even if you don't exercise, you can still gain many benefits from proper foam rolling. The key word here is "proper" as many people who have tried foam rolling and have subsequently given it up were simply not doing it correctly and therefore not seeing any benefit.

Unfortunately many books, videos and guides have been written with incorrect foam rolling techniques that can actually do more harm than good. Rest assured, however, that the methods provided in this book are tried and true methods, tested and approved by athletes, runners, bodybuilders and trainers. The exercises presented herein are easily learned and mastered and you will notice an immediate improvement in your muscle tone and joint range of motion.

Once you have mastered the foam roller, you can even take what you learned and help others to incorporate the foam roller into their routine, and you will be equipped to not only know how to do these exercises, but you can explain WHY these rolling techniques help and how they help. In other words, once you have read through this book a few times and mastered the techniques herein, you may consider yourself an expert on foam rolling. You may even want to start a class in your local gym, helping others learn the awesome benefits to foam rolling.

It is my sincerest wishes that you find the information in this book to be life as life changing as many have. I have written this book to help you change your life, through the power of self-myofascial release, by increasing your circulation, range of motion and blood flow, you should not only increase your mobility and feel better, but you will be adding years to your life, and not just years, but healthy years. So without further ado... let's start learning about foam rolling and be on our way to a better healthier life!

# A BRIEF HISTORY OF FOAM ROLLING

There has been major changes in the attitude toward injury prevention and treatment. Massage, Muscle Activation (MAT), Active Release Therapy (ART) and such have been getting much more attention as viable therapies for injured athletes. The isokinetic injury care of the eighties has given way to more hands-on soft tissue care with physical therapists using "soft tissue mobilization" (which is just a fancy way of saying "massage") and Muscle Activation as a more superior means of therapy and many chiropractors using Active Release Therapy to ease pain in the lower back.

Basically, massages have become the "in thing" in order to help heal poor aching muscles, but the problem with massages is that they are quite cost prohibitive. I mean, who doesn't want a personal massage therapist at their beck and call? But then, who can afford it, other than professional athletes and the absurdly rich. That's where foam rollers come in. You could say foam rollers are the poor man's massage therapist.

Physical Therapist Mike Clark is credited with first exposing athletic and physical therapy communities to the foam roller and to what he termed "self-myofascial release".

Clarke, in his early manuals, presented us with a means by which we can achieve a professional type of message without having to pay hundreds of dollars, and best of all we can do it ourselves. His early manuals included photos of techniques that one can use to achieve amazing results by using a simple foam roller. The techniques were extremely simple and virtually self-explanatory. These first photos began a trend that is now sweeping across the country and shows no sign of subsiding.

Clarke's initial recommendations for foam rolling was not self-massage, but more of an acupuncture technique. Basically, athletes were simply instructed to use the roller to apply pressure to certain sensitive areas of the muscles, defined as trigger points.

As massage fell out of favor, mostly due to the prohibitive costs, in the mid 1980's, such techniques as ultrasound and electrical stimulation became more popular, as trainers and therapists could use these techniques to treat more athletes and clients easily and quickly. However, for elite athletes such as track and field athletes and swimmers, a disdain for this modality approach and an attraction to massage still existed.

Slowly, the idea that manipulating soft tissue helped athletes to stay healthier and to get healthier faster caught on in the performance world.

The use of foam rollers progressed from an acupressure type approach to a self-massage approach. The roller is now used to apply longer more sweeping strokes to the long muscle groups in order to loosen tight muscles and heal micro-tares, such that occur with regular high impact exercises.

# WHAT IS
# SELF-MYOFASCIAL RELEASE?

Self-Myofascial Release is a self-massage technique where you apply pressure on a different muscles in order to release tension and improve range of movement and muscle performance.

"Myo" is the Greek word for Muscle and "Fascia" is a thin, tough, elastic type of connective tissue that wraps most structures within the human body, including muscle.

Fascia is made up of collagen fibers tightly packed together in a parallel pattern and is ubiquitous in your body linking your muscles together and providing support, stability and shape. Fascia resides in a gel-like material, called "ground substance" or "extrafibrillar matrix" that provides cushioning.

The soft Fascia tissue can become restricted due to overuse, which results in pain, muscle tension and diminished blood flow. Although fascia and its corresponding muscle are the main targets of myofascial release, other tissue may be addressed as well, including other connective tissue.

Self-myofascial release is simply the use of self-massage to release the tension in your myofascia system. Self-Myofascial Release is also known as Self Myofascial Trigger Point Therapy or Self Myofascial Trigger Point Release.

The exact phrase "myofascial release" was coined by Robert Ward, in the 1960s. Ward, along with physical therapist John Barnes, are considered the two primary founders of Myofascial Release.

During strenuous exercises or activities such as lifting heavy things or poor posture or simply overdoing it in the gym, the fascia experiences what is known as "micro-trauma" where your fascia tissue becomes tougher and less flexible, due to your body's own protective mechanism, much like your skin will create a scar or scab to protect itself.

What ends up happening is that micro-tears in the fascia will form and if these tears don't heal properly, the fascia tissue ends up stuck together. This is a condition known as an "adhesion". The trauma also causes the ground substance to solidify, which makes it much less elastic. These damaged areas in your myofascia are known as "Restricted Tissue Barriers".

As the fascia becomes tighter and develops adhesions, the underlying muscles movement will be restricted which will result in reduced flexibility, reduced range of motion and muscle aches and pains.

The fascia adhesions can also restrict your nerves and blood vessels, resulting in reduced neuromuscular efficiency (that is the connection between your brain and muscles) and ischemic (reduction in blood supply) issues. This will cause even greater pain due to the fascia adhesions restricting your nerves.

So how does self-myofascial release work to heal this damage to your myofascia system? Basically by using a foam roller you are able to put pressure on the sore and restricted tissue barriers. By applying tension, the tension will slowly be released, and your body will gradually be restored to its normal state.

The sustained pressure brought about through self-myofascial release helps to break down the adhesions in your fascia, which results in softer, more flexible, fascia tissue. This is what improves your muscle flexibility and movement. It also helps you by taking pressure off of the nerves trapped by adhesions, thus relieving pain and improving blood circulation to the soft tissues.

# CHOOSING THE RIGHT TYPE OF FOAM ROLLER

When foam rollers first came out, they were pretty much all the same, three foot pieces of white foam 6-inches in diameter. If you sent someone out to buy you a foam roller, all you had to tell them was you needed a foam roller and that's what they would get. There wasn't any question about what color or what length or how soft. There was no question of which one was the right one for you, but this has changed. Now, if you google "foam roller" on the internet, you'll get a plethora of colors, textures and lengths and materials.

Getting the right foam roller, especially when first starting out, is important if you want to get the full benefit of self-myofascial release. If you start out with the wrong roller, you may find it too painful to use and may discontinue foam rolling before you discover the awesome benefits of its continuing use. While it's true that foam rolling can (and in some cases should) be a little painful when first starting out, usually the discomfort is only minor and lasts only for a few minutes.

Choose a standard, white foam roller if you are just starting out. This is usually 3 feet long and 6 inches in diameter. The white foam roller is the easiest and gentlest of the foam rollers and can be used by just about anyone. White rollers are the softest, followed by blue or green rollers of medium density and black foam rollers, which are the firmest. White foam rollers are often made of a piece of polyethylene foam and they are the least dense, so they will allow some movement between the muscles, bones and the roller. A white foam roller will produce less pressure and less pain.

After you have been doing foam rolling for a while, you might want to move onto a medium, lightly colored foam roller for a medium amount of massage pressure. These foam rollers are usually blue or green and are made from closed cell polyethylene foam or EVA foam. They provide a bit more resistance, which in turn provides a more vigorous message.

Once you have become very experienced in foam rolling, you might want to consider a black foam roller. Although most black foam rollers are also made of polyethylene foam, they are closed cell and manufactured under high heat, making them smoother, denser and less porous. These will provide you with much more resistance for a deeper message.

If you use your roller every day (which you should), you should also consider the denser black foam roller or EVA roller, because they are much more durable. The White and colored foam rollers made of polyethylene (open celled) materials can warp over time with repeated use. However, if you do desire a softer foam roller, you can usually find a good brand guaranteed not to warp.

Besides the foam rollers listed above, there are even firmer, more advanced rollers available which are good for those who have been foam rolling a while and desire a more solid, less resistant roller. Though most people are fine with the black roller, some need that extra vigorous deep down body message.

If you have been foam rolling for a good while, and find the foam just isn't doing it for you, you might think about trying "The Grid" roller. The grid has a hard, hollow core which is wrapped in EVA foam, which makes it firmer than traditional the traditional foam rollers. This roller is designed with proprietary Distrodensity zones. The three dimensional surface has a variety of widths to replicate the feeling of a massage therapist's hands. The grid also comes in the larger 26-inch length and is 5-inches in diameter.

A step up from the grid would be the Rumble Roller. This is definitely not your first choice for foam rolling, as it can be very painful if you are not used to rolling. While the foam rollers listed above simply compress your soft tissue, the Rumble Roller actually manipulates this tissue (like a vigorous message therapist might do). The surface of this roller contains specially designed bumps that are firm, but flexible, much like the thumbs of a massage therapist. As you roll over the top of the Rumble Roller, the bumps continuously knead the contours of your body, stretching the muscle and fascia in multiple directions. This is excellent for getting into hamstrings and gastrocnemius muscles that may be sore as well as helping to correct Iliotibial band issues and piriformis pain.

Another thing you will need to decide on is the size of your foam roller. Most foam rollers are 6 inches in diameter (though some come in 5"). The length of the rollers however range from 12 inches to 36 inches. If you plan to use your roller on your back, a 26-inch to 36-inch foam roller would probably be your best choice. The longer rollers allow you to roll with it at a right angle to your back giving your back full support while you roll. The smaller, 12-inch roller is the best choice if you plan on transporting your roller, as it is compact and easily transported, but it does not provide as much support for your back. I recommend you purchase several different sizes of rollers, for different rolling techniques, perhaps a small (12-inch) roller, a medium sized (18 to 20-inch roller) and a longer (26 to 36-inch) roller.

Of course, another major decision to make when buying your first foam roller (or rollers) is how much you want to spend on it. A standard 12 inch white foam roller will usually be the least expensive, costing under $15.00. A black foam roller is considered a professional grade roller and might cost upwards of $30.

EVA foam rollers are becoming much more popular these days. These are usually the green rollers and are moderately firm with a more comfortable surface that is warm to the touch. They are much more durable than polyethylene foam rollers but will cost you up to $45.

There are so many different brands, types, colors and varieties to choose from, you may find it hard to decide on which is the best one for you. In order to make this a little easier on you, I've listed below some of the most popular, which I feel are the best bet for quality and durability.

**Perform Better Elite Molded Foam Rollers**

The Perform Better Elite Molded Foam roller keeps its shape very well and provides a nice solid surface to roll on. This is the most durable roller out there, in my opinion, especially for heavier people (over 180 pounds). You can use this roller over and over without seeing any decrease in quality. Most roller gurus agree, if you want a good firm roller that keeps its shape and will last a long time, this is the best choice.

## Foam Roller Plus

If you are looking for something that's a little less firm, you'll want to go for the Foam Roller Plus. The problem with most of the softer foam rollers is that they tend to flatten out over time, which means you end up having to replace them more often. However, the Foam Roller Plus has a rigid PVC core with a softer foam coating, which helps make it more comfortable while still retaining its shape. It also has a removable washable neoprene cover which makes it ideal for those situations where multiple people might use it.

## EVA Foam Rollers

As mentioned above, EVA foam rollers are made of closed cell foam, and therefore keep their shape much better than the open-celled soft polyethylene rollers. However, for heavier people (over 200 pounds) they tend to also get crushed after repeated use. Another downside is that they are a bit more expensive than the standard Foam rollers.

## The Grid Foam Roller

This foam roller is quite similar to the Foam Roller Plus in that it is a rigid PVC roll with a soft outer cover. It is even the same price as the Foam Roller Plus. The only real difference as far as I can see between The Grid and the Foam Roller Plus is that The Grid is slightly less resistant and the Foam Roller plus has the removable neoprene cover.

# THE EXERCISES

Now that we have learned what self-myofascial release is and how it works, what the different types of foam rollers are and how they work and how to choose the best roller for you, it's time to learn how to use the rollers for maximum benefit.

If you go through the internet, you will find a plethora of exercises available for foam rolling, some of these are excellent and some of them, to be quite frank, are useless or even worse, they may be dangerous. If you've tried foam rolling on your own, you may have noticed little or no improvement, or you may have experienced pain that caused you to turn away from foam rolling.

Of course, there will be some initial pain when you start your rolling regiment, but this is about the same amount of pain you should feel from getting any deep message and should ease up as you continue to smooth out and release the fascial material that causes your muscles to feel knotted up. One of the main things you should keep in mind, especially when first starting out with foam rolling is to take it slow and easy and use a soft pliable (white) roller, so as not to aggravate the tight muscles even further.

In this chapter I'll touch on the most effective exercises for each of the muscle groups. I wouldn't suggest you do all of these exercises at once, but work on those muscles that are giving you the most pain. You can also do some exercises one day and work on different groups of muscles the next day, and so on.

Of course, before starting any kind of exercise regimen, it's always advisable to talk to your doctor to be sure you're up to it. More than likely, though, your doctor will be more than enthusiastic about your self-myofascial release exercises.

## Neck Muscles

Foam rolling on your neck will help to facilitate postural alignment and provide pain relief by focusing on the tight spots within the neck muscles. You should be very careful to go slowly when treating any neck pain or when first starting out, as overdoing it may cause strain to your neck and may even cause injury. A few moments a day is really all you need to loosen those neck muscles.

To start off this exercise, you should lie flat on your back with the foam roller placed under your neck. Keep your head up and lift your hips off the floor slowly until your weight is on your neck muscles. This is one exercise where there really is very little rolling involved, but the object is to slowly move the neck back and forth and side to side to find the tight or sensitive spots. When a tight spot is found, keep the pressure on that spot until gradually it releases (but no longer than a minute).

Once you have released most (or hopefully all) of the tight spots on the back of your neck, turn over on your side and once again slowly lift your hips until most of your weight is on the side of your neck. Be sure to only put as much pressure on your neck as is comfortable and if there is too much pain stop immediately. Don't do any rolling, just allow your neck to remain on the roller for a minute to relieve knotted muscles and tension. Turn over and do the same for the other side of your neck.

## Upper Back

The upper back (or thoracic) area is an area that often holds tension. When we get stressed, we tend to hold our breath which lifts the scapulae (shoulder blades), trapezius (upper part of the shoulders) and neck. This tension leads to upper back pain, imbalance and poor posture

While performing the following upper back exercises, it is important to breathe deeply, as this will help to increase the release desired as well as keeping you more relaxed. Deep breathing is necessary to maintaining healthy oxygen flow to your muscles and is also necessary to keep your brain healthy and focused.

To start this exercise, position the foam roller directly beneath your shoulder blades. Support your head with your hands, keeping your knees bent and your feet flat on the floor.

Gently start rolling the foam roller toward your head, using your feet to control your motion. Pause the roller whenever you reach a tight or sore spot, and by using deep breathing, allow that spot to be pressed down on the roller, using very small movements until the tension subsides. Continue rolling up toward your neck, then pause and roll down until your reach the middle of your back. Continue rolling up and down until you have rolled away all tension from your upper back.

It may take some time, but eventually you will be able to guide the roller exactly where your tension lies, by moving slowly up and down and slightly changing position from each side, so that each portion of the fascia has been addressed and all adhesions have been released.

**Lower Back**

The Upper Back exercise above will also help relieve much of the strain on your lower back as well. However, in order to touch on the smaller muscles in your lower back, you will want to transition from the upper back to the lower back, by starting with the upper back exercise, then slowly rolling toward your buttocks, holding pressure on any tight spots you feel right above your buttocks.

You should ease from side to side rolling from the middle of your back toward the hips then back up. You should immediately feel a release in your lower back if you are doing this properly. If you are feeling any kind of strain when doing this, you should try to reposition your hands toward your legs, holding your thighs above the knees.

This will take some pressure off of the back. Don't overdue the lower back exercise or you may end up stretching the muscles and straining them rather than releasing them. Remember to stop at any spot that feels tight and allow your muscles to sink into the roller until the tightness has been released.

**Hip Flexors**

The Hip Flexors are a group of muscles that control the hip joint, allowing it to rotate and move the knees upward. In actuality, there are quite a few muscles that work toward flexing the hip, but there are two muscles specifically that are referred to as hip flexors. The Illiosoas group of muscles consists of the Psoas muscil and Iliacus. Both of these muscles are attached to the femur, with the psoas muscle attached to the lower back and Iliacus attached to the hipbone.

Because the hip joint is extremely mobile, these muscles are high susceptible to injury and stiffness. Sitting for long periods of time without periods of stretching can cause the hip flexors to become very tight and cause pain and stiffness. The reason for this stiffness and tightness is due to the way the muscles are contracted when in a sitting position.

Hip Flexor exorcises can help to relieve this tension in both the hip and the buttocks, as the hip flexors muscles are in close proximity to the gluteal muscles. Once you have performed this foam rolling technique a few times, you should find it much easier to sit for longer period of times without feeling that tensions in your back, hips and buttocks. However, it is strongly advised to those who do have to sit for long period of times to stand up and stretch several times at regular intervals to keep the hip flexors (and the gluteal muscles) from becoming stiff and sore in the first place.

There are two different exercises that are recommended with the roller to help to smooth out and release the tension in your hip flexors.

The first exercise helps you to release the gluteal muscles and is performed by lying face up with the foam roller directly under one side of your buttocks. Keep your legs straight and support you upper body with your elbows. Now slowly roll back and forth over the foam roller, making sure to keep your hips and buttocks relaxed. Keep rolling for about a minute, then do the other side.

The next exercise is done in a similar way, except that you will lie on your side and rest your hip on the roller. You will, again, be holding your body weight on your elbow as you slowly roll your hip up and down over the foam roller for about a minute on each side. As you do these exercises be sure to breathe slowly and make the rolls as smoothly as possible. At first it may be painful, but slowly as you do the exercise, you should fill a release of tension in both your hip flexor muscles as well as gluteal muscles.

## IT Band

The Iliotibial (or IT) Band is a very strong, thick band of fibrous tissue running along the leg on the outside. The IT band runs from the hip, along the thigh, attaching to the edge of the tibia (shin bone) just below the knee. This band provides stability to the outside of the knee joint, working with the quadriceps (thigh muscles) during movement.

When the IT band is overused or injured, it may become inflamed, in which case Iliotibial band syndrome may occur. This is particularly common in runners, cyclists, and people who participate in other aerobic activities. The IT band becomes irritated, due to repeated use during running and other activities in which its stabilizer function comes into constant play.

IT Band Syndrome can be very painful, and is felt mostly on the outside (lateral) of the knee and/or on the lower thigh. It is often most pronounced when climbing stairs and rising from a sitting position.

While foam rolling the IT band may be painful at first, especially in those dealing with moderate to severe IT Band Syndrome, it is probably one of the most useful self-myofascial exercises you will perform with the foam roller.

Begin by lying on your side, with the roller placed just below your hip. Bend the top leg in front of you over your bottom leg, and place the foot of our top leg on the floor. This will help you maintain your balance as well as allowing you to adjust how much weight is applied to the roller by placing more or less weight on your foot.

If you want more pressure you can keep your top leg perpendicular to your bottom leg. This will place much more pressure on the roller, so it may be much more painful.

Using your hands for support, roll from the hip down toward the knees, pausing whenever you reach any tight or painful spots. Once you have reached just above the knee, roll back up toward the hip. Do this two or three times until you have reached all of the tight spots, then turn on your other side and repeat it.

**Calf Stretch Exercise**

The calf muscle group consists of the gastrocnemius muscle and the soleus muscle. These muscles could gradually tighten when running and may end up becoming more painful; over time, especially when one neglects stretching or self-myofascial workouts before running.

If your calves are too tight, the muscles on the front of your thigh (quadriceps muscles) have to work harder to extend your knee. This can overload the patellar tendon and lead to knee pain.

To help loosen the calf and relieve tightness, start by placing the roller underneath your right calf with your left leg, kneed bent, placed to the side of the roller. Roll the calf muscle very slowly over the roller from the ankle to just below the knee. When you encounter and tenderness or tightness in the muscle, you should hold that position until you feel the tightness begin to t release. Keep rolling for about a minute to a minute and an half and then do the same thing with your other leg.

If you need to apply more pressure, you can place on leg on the other. Or, conversely, to apply less pressure roll both legs at once. Roll with your feet turned in and out and keep your toes flexed in order to work the entire muscle group.

## Quadriceps

The quadriceps are the group of muscles on the front of your thighs. There are four distinct muscles that make up the quadriceps muscles; the vastus intermedius, the vastus medialis, the vastus lateralis, and the rectus femoris.

When your quads (as they are often called) contract, they straighten your leg at the knee joint. Since the quadriceps also extend over the kneecap (patella), the quads help to keep your kneecap in the right position. Injury to the quad could result in a dislocated knee cap, and if you have arthritis the quadriceps may stop working properly. This may result in a condition known as Patella Femoral Stress syndrome, which is when the quads become unable to help the kneecap to keep its position. Your quads might be weakened in cases due to spinal cord injury or paresis (a condition caused by stroke). Lower back pain may also cause a pinched nerve that might weaken the quadriceps.

Your quadriceps help you straighten your knees, which is especially essential when rising from a sitting position. They are are also a major muscle group responsible for walking up and down stairs as well as being essential for walking and running.

Weakness in the quads may result in an inability to keep ones balance as well as the inability to walk straight, or normal. As you can see, this group of muscles is very important to your day to day life, not just in professional athletes but in everybody.

Luckily keeping your quads released and conditioned is one of the easiest foam roller exercises, and the results can help keep your knees and legs healthy over a much longer period of time.

Simply place the roller under the thigh you wish to release, right below the hip and, using your hands to balance you, start rolling from the hip down to the knee and back up again. Do this several time for both thighs.

If you need more pressure, you can roll both legs on the roller and place your body in a position as if you were ready to do some pushups, in this manner you can apply as much pressure (by focusing your weight on the roller) as you want.

If you want less pressure, just keep one leg off of the roller, using he foot to support some of your body weight.

## Glutes and Hamstrings

Sitting for long periods of time may lead to the gluteal muscles (Glutes) atrophying through constant pressure and disuse. This could result in lower back pain as well as difficulty with movements, such as standing from a sitting position and climbing stairs that naturally require the gluteal muscles.

The hamstring muscle group consists of three separate muscles; the semitendinosus, semimembranosus and biceps femoris. Hamstring strains most commonly occur in the biceps femoris muscle (at the point where the muscle joins the tendon), but might also occur higher in the semimembranosus muscle. During sprinting the first type of strain is more likely to occur, while the latter is usually due to stretching.

Sprinting related hamstring injuries often feel worse but recover more quickly, whereas stretch related hamstring strains can take longer to heal die the face that the injury is more likely to the tendon, where there is lesser blood flow.

If you have ever pulled a hamstring, you know how painful this can be and how long it takes a pulled hamstring muscle to heal. This exercise is essential to keep your hamstring muscles from getting tight in the first place, which is the primary cause of all hamstring injury.

This exercise will loosen both your hamstrings and your glutes, simultaneously.

Start this exercise by sitting on the roller with the soft, meaty part of your buttock directly on top of the roller. Slowly roll back and forth with a slight side to side movement to release the tight spots, starting from the top of your buttocks slowly rolling down the back of your legs toward your knee, while working the hamstrings. As you work downwards stop whenever you feel a tight or sore spot, and allow the pressure to relax the muscles. You can increase or decrease the pressure by using only one leg, or using both legs at the same time. Roll with your feet turned in and out to cover the entire muscle group.

## Soles of the Feet

The American College of Sports and Medicine estimates that the average adult takes between 5,000 and 10,000 steps per day. Most of this activity is borne by the muscles and ligaments of the foot.

Arch pain is most commonly felt as discomfort under the long arch of the foot. It can vary in severity, and can be characterized by pain in the arch of the foot on weight bearing after rest or gradual onset during the day. The structure most often involved is the plantar fascia, the band of tissue that supports the arch of the foot.

The plantar fascia ligament is located along the sole of your foot. This ligament is made of up fascia that stretch from the heel and branches out across the arch through the ball of the foot toward the toes. This is the ligament that gives you the bounce and spring in your normal daily activities.

In the case of Plantar Fasciitis, the plantar fascia is stretched more than it should be which ends up resulting in small tears in the fascia. Every time you flex your foot, those tendons, ligaments, and tissue move and when they are inflamed, every movement hurts.

Luckily there is a quick and easy remedy to help keep your muscles and tendons free of stress and strain, using your friendly roller. There are several different ways you can use your foam roller to relieve foot stress and keep your feet healthy and happy.

One of the simplest and easiest ways is to sit down on a comfortable chair, with the roller beneath your feet. Starting from the middle of the foot, slowly roll your foot up toward the toes, stopping just before you reach your toes, then roll back toward the heel. Continue to work back and forth and moving slightly from side to side on each foot several times. You should immediately feel much of the strain on your feet ease.

Another method is to perform the same exercise as stipulated above, but do it from a sanding position while using something to stead yourself. You can do this with one foot at a time or both feet, but be very cautious to have something to hold on to, and only try this if you have a good sense of balance as it is very easy to fall right on your Gluteus Maximus.

# WHY DOES IT HURT?

One of the most common questions I am asked by people just getting started in foam rolling is, "Why does it hurt?" or "Is it supposed to hurt this much?". The answer to this question depends on how much hurt we are talking about. Some pain is to be expected, as you are loosening and releasing tight muscles and joints. If you want an example of what we are talking about, make a fist and hold it for about two minutes, tight as you can. Then slowly release your fist. You will notice that this is a bit painful when you release your fist. Your fascial material, muscles, joints and tendons are much like your tightened fist, especially if they have been in a contracted position for a long period of time, so when you first start rolling, there will be that same type of pain or discomfort you felt when releasing your fist.

There is no cause for alarm, as this is normal and the more you release your tight muscles and joints, the less pain you will feel over time. The first few times, however, will more than likely result in some discomfort and pain. It should be stressed however, that this pain should be only minor and if you are feeling a great deal of pain, you may have a sprain or strain that should be treated by a doctor or therapist before you continue your foam rolling routine.

How much pain is too much pain? If it is almost bringing tears to your eyes, then it is probably too much pain. It shouldn't be so painful that you can hardly take it, but rather a minor pain, such as you would experience unclenching your fist after holding it tight for a couple minutes. Each person experiences pain differently and what may seem extremely painful to one person might seem only minor to another. Therefore, it's really hard to exactly pinpoint how much pain is too much pain. If you can get through your rolling session, with some pain, then you should be okay, but if it's just too painful to continue you might seek medical advice. Once you roll on a regular basis, the pain and discomfort should dissipate to where you are feeling only a release with no pain at all.

Another thing to keep in mind is that if you are not properly doing the exercises outlined in this book, there is a chance you may actually pull a muscle or sprain something, which is why it is very important to do these exercises exactly as outline. Don't try to improvise, at least not until you have gotten the hang of it and can do so safely (by gauging the amount of strain on your joints and muscles) and stay away from the overwhelming amount of rolling exercises and programs found online, as many of these exercises can actually cause more harm than good. Our exercises in this book are tried and proven and are guaranteed to cause no strain or stress on key muscle groups.

If you've ever received a massage from a professional massage therapist, you'll know that there is going to be some pain involved when releasing tight muscles, but after a while that pain will eventually subside and be replaced with a feeling of great release and relaxation. It should be the same thing with self-myofascial release. There will be an initial pain as your muscles loosen, but it shouldn't last more than one or two session, after which you will feel only the soothing release of any tight muscles.

I would like to stress once more, however, if there is extreme pain in any of your joints or muscles, you should immediately consult a doctor or therapist to determine if there is any underlying damage, before continuing with foam rolling. Even though foam rolling is one of the safest methods of releasing tight muscles and reducing painful inflammation that comes from rigorous exercise, if there is torn ligaments or other problems, it could further damage the tissue by applying pressure to the affected area, so please see your doctor if you experience excruciating pain while rolling, or if your pain does not go away within a couple of sessions, as this could be an indication of a more serious problem.

# TRIGGER POINT THERAPY

One of the main reasons you might feel pain during your rolling session is due to something called a "trigger point". Myofascial trigger points are aggravated spots in fascia tissue with substantial swellings in small bands of muscle fibers. There is little actual scientific or medical research to date on trigger points and therefore some disagreement within the medical community on how to treat myofascial trigger point pain, or even the cause of such pain.

In their medical textbook, "Myofascial Pain and Dysfunction: The Trigger Point Manual", Drs. Janet travel and David Simons define trigger points as tiny contraction knots that develop in the muscle due to overwork or injury.

The actual muscle fiber that is doing all of this contracting is called the sarcomere, a microscopic unit in the muscle. When the the two parts of sarcomere come together to interlock it causes an extremely minute contraction. If a million sarcomere interlocked in your muscle, it might cause a slight twitch.

Normally, sarcomeres act as pumps in the body, as the muscle works these microscopic fibers contract and relax to help in blood circulation. Trigger points occur when overstimulated sarcomeres are unable to release from an interlocked state. This in turn causes the muscles to become starved for oxygen while the buildup of metabolisms irritate the trigger point. This in turn causes the trigger point to send out pain signals to the brain through the muscle fibers being affected.

The problem with these signals is that, with trigger point, we have referred pain, which basically means that trigger points will send their pain to some other site, so that we may have pains in other parts of our bodies and, instead of actually paying attention to the trigger site, we try to treat that area of the body.

A trigger point can cause headaches, neck pain, lower back pain, jaw pain and may be mistaken as tennis elbow or Carpal Tunnel Syndrome. The pain might also be the source of pain in areas of the body that may be misdiagnosed as arthritis, tendinitis or bursitis.

A trigger point may be found in the upper back that, when pressed, may cause referred pain in the neck, whereupon the neck may act as a satellite trigger point, further causing pain in the head or eyes. This pain may be a sharp pain or it may be dull and throbbing.

The trigger point model says that unexplained pain usually radiate from small local tenderness outward toward the broader areas which may, in fact, be quite distant from the original trigger point. Many therapists have found that certain patterns of pain can be attributed to and traced to certain trigger points in disparate locations about the body. When the trigger point is pressed (or compressed) local tenderness, referred pain or twitching will usually be the response. It should be noted that this twitching is not to be confused with spasms, where a muscle spasm effect a larger group of muscles, the twitching will be small localized around the actual trigger point.

The actual term "trigger point" did not come into use until 1942, when Dr. Janet Travell used this term to describe certain clinical findings that had the following criteria:

The problem with trigger points is that medical doctors, physicians and practitioners, as well as actual physical therapists are not always aware of the trigger point and may treat pain as another possible condition, due to the very limited understand of myofascial trigger points today. The good news, however, is that the medical community is starting to become more aware and thankfully many people are learning not only the source of their pain, but the awesome power the foam roller has in relieving trigger points and reducing the pain felt due to these trigger points.

If you go through the exercises in this book, you'll find that often there will be very sore spots on your muscles that make the rolling seem more painful than in other places. The trick with myofascial trigger points is in finding the trigger point and focusing on that trigger point with the roller, gently back and forth as if kneading bread to get the lumps out. You will know you've found a trigger point when you feel pain radiating outward from that point, especially in whole muscle groups, simply by pushing on that single point. You will also notice the point is harder, often with a lump or a knot.

Traditionally, with a typical trigger point, one would see a professional to have them message these point breaking up the sarcomeres and improving blood circulation to that point. With the invention of Foam Rollers, however, and myofascial release therapy, we can work our own trigger points even more effectively, and much less expensive as well.

You will note on all of the exercises in this book that if you come across a particularly tight or sore spot, it's suggested you focus the roller gently on that spot, until the pain dissipates. When you hit a particularly aggressive trigger point, you may be tempted to quit rolling as the pain will be much more pronounced, but don't give into that temptation. Simply ease into the spot, putting less pressure then slowly rolling your way toward more pressure until you feel the tension and pain decreasing. After a short while, as your muscle fibers are getting more oxygen, and the blood flow increases, you will find a release of those tight muscles and often even notice pain from other areas disappearing as well.

Finding those trigger points and releasing them is vital to helping your muscles remain healthy. Some preliminary research even shows that these trigger point may be a leading cause of fibromyalgia and other serious painful conditions, so taking care of them now may help avoid many conditions in the future caused by muscular oxygen deprivation and metabolic buildups originating with trigger points. A regular foam rolling regimen may go a long ways to preventing many age-related ailments as well, caused by tight muscles as well as improper oxygen flow in the muscles.

# FOAM ROLLING
# FOR RUNNERS

Many runners have found foam rolling to be an important part of their regimen, even healthy runners who feel no pain or discomfort after running. The main benefit of foam rolling for runners has to do mostly with the mobility of the fascia. If the fascia is not properly mobile the fibers may become cross linked and bind themselves to our nerves and muscles, which impedes normal movement and may cause pain over time.

Most runners will perform stretching exercises in order to keep their muscles from tightening up, but recent research has found that stretching may not be enough. A study published in the Journal of Sport Rehabilitation (January 2014) found that there was a much increased range of motion in the hip joint after rolling the hamstring, then with stretching exercises alone. It is postulated that this is due to an increase blood flow and an increase in intramuscular temperature. Both of these are necessary to help the elastic properties of the muscle.

The above mentioned study suggests that stretching prior to exercise is may not only be unbeneficial, but may even cause injuries. Many experts are now suggesting that stretching should only be performed after the run, as the muscles are relaxing and returning to their normal positions and lengths. The study also suggested that it might be of a greater benefit to perform self-myofascial release preceding the post exercise stretch.

It is important to understand how fascia is constantly being created and renewed in our body. As we put stress on our own body, especially through exercises such as running, that stress will affect how the body is forming those fibers which may cause pain and problems in mobility. By utilizing the foam rolling techniques outlined in this book we can keep trigger points and scar tissue from forming by breaking up those tissues within the muscle and the fascia. This will allow our tissue the proper mobility and help with normal function and motion.

As you continue with Self-Myofascial release exercises, you muscles will become more flexible and perform within the normal range of motion. This will enable them to be more productive and produce more power, due to the elastic energy inherent within them. As a muscle stretches it stores more energy the more it stretches and the more stored energy it has the greater the force it will be able to produce. If there is less flexibility in the muscle, there will be a reduced elasticity (or stretch), which in turn provides a reduced range of motion, less stored energy and a decrease in force output.

If you are a runner, combining foam rolling with proper stretching can help your muscles to perform at their peak performance level which will help you to achieve a greater standard of performance than you may have thought possible.

# INCORPORATING THE FOAM ROLLER INTO YOUR YOGA ROUTINE

I have received quite a few questions dealing with Yoga and foam rolling. Many people know about foam rollers and how great they are in helping with many different fitness routines. Most people, however, don't realize how much the foam roller fits right into many different yoga routines, helping to increase range of motion and flexibility as well as providing muscle tissues with increased blood flow and oxygen.

While many people think that yoga is all about stretching, Yoga is much more than this, it is creating a balance in the body by developing both strength and flexibility. One way this is achieved is by placing your body in a variety of positions, or poses. Your practice (or your individual experience with yoga) will always change, it is not to be static. That's not to say that the poses will change, but your experience with yoga will change, always evolving. By adding foam rolling to your practice, you will find that you will achieve an even greater balance and feeling wellness from your head to your feet.

Many fitness trainers and enthusiasts noticed that when they started with foam rolling, many of the exercises looked very similar to many yoga positions and sessions. If you have done any type of yoga, you may have noticed the similarity in those exercises listed in this book. Because so many yoga poses are similar to foam roller exercises, it is much easier to adjust your yoga sessions to include the foam roller as an integral part of your yoga practice.

Below, I have listed a few yoga positions and exercises that can be greatly enhanced using the foam roller. This is just some ideas, but as you do your yoga postures, you will no doubt find many other uses for the foam roller in your yoga practice.

## Plank Position

Instead of resting your forearms on the floor, you can use the roller instead. In this manner you can push back and forth with your arms, thus incorporating an added level of balance and control to the plank position.

## Pike Position

From the chaturanga pose you can place your ankles on the roller, then roll up into the pike position and then back to the chaturanga pose. This will help you to increase your lower leg muscle and mobility.

## Bridge Position

As you move your body into the bridge position, position your lower spine on your roller. You can then pull your knees up to your chest and rotate the knees and legs in a circular mostion, which will help to massage your lower spine, relieving tension from the lower back.

**Downward facing dog**

While you are in the downward facing dog position, you can utilize the roller by placing your thighs on the roller and move down to the upward facing dog. From this position, allow your body to move into a low plank while rolling the front of the thighs, moving from the plank to the upward facing dog and back into the plank position. You can move into the side facing plank and roll the outer thighs, as well.

These are just a few examples of how you can utilize the roller with your yoga, and there are probably dozens if not hundreds of other ways of using that roller to enhance your yoga practice. If you already have a good practice set up, you'll find that it's almost second nature to incorporate the roller into them, to add balancing, toning and control to your practice.

On the other side of the coin, you may find while performing the exercises already outlined in this book, you can also incorporate Yoga into your roller exercises, as many of the roller positions will mirror many of your yoga positions to some degree. Just allow yourself to be creative, but remember not to overdo it. With Yoga, in many cases you are stretching your body to extremes, but by incorporating the roller, you allow your body to stretch, release and massage many points, thus helping you to not only enhance the exercises but to decrease the likelihood of accidental sprains and tears to your facial tissue.

# ROLLING BACK THE YEARS

This may sound like an exaggerated claim, but foam rolling may actually help to not only make you feel younger and more vital, but can be an extreme benefit to actually slowing the aging process and helping you to live a longer, healthier life. While it hasn't been "scientifically proven" there are many theories why this is true, which we will cover in this chapter.

One effect of aging is sore muscles, limited mobility and certain muscle and tendon issues such as arthritis and bursitis that tend to creep up on us as we age. Some doctors are prone to saying "you're just getting older", suggesting these conditions are normal and we should just accept them as part of our aging process. This is hogwash!

If you recall from our previous chapter on trigger point therapy, there are certain microfibers then can get "knotted" over time, called sarcomeres. As these fibers continue to contract without releasing, they begin to pile up causing poor circulation and depriving our muscles of oxygen necessary to keep them healthy and working properly. If left unattended, as we age these knots or trigger points become more and more pronounced and we tend to find more aches and pains setting in, until eventually those muscles no longer function properly. Theoretically, this could very well be the cause of many ailments we face in our latter years, such as arthritic pain, lower and upper back pain, leg pain, etc.

Low or poor blood circulation can cause many different health issues, including heart issues that may lead to death. Utilizing the roller exercises in this book will help you to actually increase your blood circulation by breaking up those tight areas where your fascial tissue may be knotted. Improving blood circulation improves oxygen flow to your entire body. All of our organs need a good supply of oxygen in order to function properly, and as we age these organs may end up having serious issues if they have consistently been not receiving the proper supply of oxygen.

If you are young now, then it's the perfect time to start rolling, as this will keep your muscles working proper, thus adding years to your mobility. If you keep up with your exercises daily, you'll be helping yourself avoid a plethora of health problems that come about through inactive muscles and poor circulation so that by the time you reach into your 60's and 70's you'll find yourself feeling healthy and vital as others fall victim to "old age".

The great news is that, if you're already "over the hill" and suffering from these ailments so often associated with old age, it's not too late to do something about it. The nice thing about foam rolling is that, unlike many exercises, most of these exercises are safe and effective, regardless of your age or condition. Of course, you will want to talk with your doctor first, but in most cases you will find that adding foam rolling to your daily regimen will be nothing but beneficial to you.

I have heard from men and women into their 80's who have raved at how foam rolling has given them a new lease on life! One woman who recently celebrated her 80th birthday had been suffering from lower hip pains that doctors had been treating by giving her pain medication, for the last 5 years. However it had been progressively getting worse and she was desperate for a cure and tired of being told it was "old age" and she should just accept it. Luckily she didn't accept this, she went out looking for answers, and she came across an article about foam rolling helping in several different joint pain therapies.

She went out and bought a foam roller and she started doing some of the exercises (listed in this book) and found that by just gently rolling on her side for 10 minutes a day, coupled with a few other easy rolling exercises, her pain started to dissipate. She eventually found that there were numerous trigger points in her lower back that was actually the root cause of her pain. In just a couple of months, this woman says she felt years younger and her family is amazed at her increased mobility and the vitality she is exhibiting. Her friends and family have commented that after she turned 80 she seems to have been turning back the clock, and is moving around like she did 20 years ago.

While not all people are going to have the same drastic results, I wanted to share this story to illustrate how much foam rollers can help both the young and the old. We don't need to listen to doctors telling us we are just getting older and we don't have to just accept it. With foam rolling you can actually roll back that clock, if you are elderly. If you are young you can slow down or stop that clock from ticking, by keeping your circulation healthy, thus keeping your body healthy.

# CONCLUSION

If you've made it all the way through this book, Congratulations! You are now on your way to being an expert in self-myofascial release.

You've learned how foam rolling came about, what exactly self-myofascial release is about and why foam rolling can really help you in keeping yourself limber with full-range of motions in your joints and muscles.

You've also learned that by utilizing your foam roller daily, you can add years to your life or take years off your life, by increasing your circulation and keeping your muscles from knotting up.

You've learned the very best exercises from the neck to the soles of the feet and not only how to do the exercises by why you should be doing the exercises as well.

You can use these exercises by themselves, or you can perform these exercises before and after training or workouts, in order to keep yourself limber and to release any adhesions inherent with most workouts.

I highly recommend, if you haven't yet checked it out, that you also start working with some yoga postures to help increase the effectiveness of your rolling. If you already are into yoga, you've learned herein how easy it is to incorporate the foam roller into many yoga poses, in order to maximize the effectiveness of the yoga routine. Yoga and Foam rolling go together quite well in helping to to keep muscles and tendons limber and keep your blood circulation at peak performance.

Eventually, once you have tried all of the exercises in this book you will develop your own regime, such as doing the upper back exercises followed by the neck exercises. You may want to incorporate several exercises a day, or simply do a different exercise each day. This is a personal choice depending on what your personal needs are and why you are doing these exercises. While some people find that doing all of the exercises in succession provides them with the most benefit, others may find that focusing on only one or two areas each day is perfect for them. Each person is unique, so you should find what works best for you and go with that.

As you progress in your rolling exercises you may even find yourself improvising and coming up with new techniques. Just remember, when you do any self-myofascial release, there should be very little pain and no strain on any muscles. If you feel you are straining, then you need to ease off and/or position yourself so that there is no strain. There will, more than likely, be some slight pain or discomfort when you first begin, but this will very quickly ease up and you will feel a release soon afterward.

Keep in mind, as well, that if or when you hit a trigger point, you may experience an increase in your pain, but as you gently and firmly focus your rolling on the trigger point, this pain will decrease and you will feel a release in both tension as well as pain. Don't stop rolling when you do encounter one of those "tender" spots that cause you pain, just ease up a little and ease into the trigger point until it is released.

Remember, by releasing trigger points, you are actually increasing the flow of blood and oxygen to your muscles and the rest of your body, which will help to not only make you feel better, but may also help to stave off many age-related illnesses that are often chalked up to "your just getting old". This is why it's very important to not give up when you feel that pain, or to avoid that area, but to work it out with the foam roller until it has eased up and your circulation has returned to normal.

I would also like to say, if your doctor just says your pains and lack of mobility is "normal" and it's just a part of aging, you might think about finding another doctor. I know many doctors will hate me for this, but there is ALWAYS a reason, a root cause to any pain or discomfort and it's just plain lazy to say it's due to old age and nothing can be done about it, but give them pills and let them deal with it.

One way to find a good doctor is when the doctor examines you, asks questions about your lifestyle, diet and exercise and offers suggestions to help you to increase your circulation, mobility and muscle tone. A great doctor would be one who suggests you get a foam roller, in my humble opinion, as this is one of the best way to reverse many muscle related ailments, as well as ailments rooted in poor circulation.

Once you have mastered the techniques found in this book, you will probably find that foam rolling is so addictive that your body will complain if you go a couple days without it. It's one of the best and easiest ways to give your body that all over massage without having to hire a professional masseuse, and of course much less expensive.

So save your money, save your muscles and save your mobility, get yourself a foam roller (if you haven't already done so) and get to feeling better, more energized and healthier through self-myofascial release.